Diets to help CYSTITIS

Cystitis is an irritating and, usually, chronic infection of the urinary system which often defies symptomatic treatment through antibiotics. Here, Ralph McCutcheon, a naturopath, osteopath, acupuncturist and kinesiologist, describes a full nutritional approach to restore the body's underlying health and to heal damaged tissue once and for all.

Diets to help
CYSTITIS

RALPH McCUTCHEON
N.D., D.O., B.Ac

Thorsons
An Imprint of HarperCollinsPublishers

Thorsons
An Imprint of HarperCollins*Publishers*
77–85 Fulham Palace Road,
Hammersmith, London W6 8JB
1160 Battery Street,
San Francisco, California 94111–1213

First published by Thorsons 1980
This edition, revised and updated, 1993
10 9 8 7 6 5 4 3 2 1

Ralph McCutcheon asserts the moral right to
be identified as the author of this work

A catalogue record for this book
is available from the British Library

ISBN 0 7225 2872 8

Phototypeset by Harper Phototypesetters Limited,
Northampton, England
Printed in Great Britain by
HarperCollinsManufacturing Glasgow

Contents

Introduction

SELF-HELP OR PROFESSIONAL HELP

In common with many medical conditions, the problem with writing a book on self-help for cystitis is to differentiate between those cases needing professional help and those which can be readily treated at home. This has been written as a guide to which treatment may be most desirable, as well as a manual on self-help.

Careful assessment of symptoms is needed to work out a suitable treatment programme, so comparative tables have been included for easy reference (see the Appendix). In most cases alternative approaches are recommended and further reference should be made to the text for guidance as to which one or combination is likely to suit you best.

TREATING THE WHOLE BODY

Always remember that a symptom, be it cystitis or a sore ear, is a reflection of the total condition of the body and the root cause of the disturbance may be apparently remote from the symptom. It does not necessarily follow that just because a symptom goes away for a while the cause has been dealt with.

The human body is a vastly complex creation, in which the well-being of each individual cell and part affects, directly or indirectly, the health of every other. The various indications given in this book cover most causes likely to be encountered, but we are all different and if nothing seems to match up to your own feelings and observations of your condition, it may be necessary to consult a skilled clinician in order to build up a picture of the causes and effects.

Cystitis tends to occur mainly in women, though men are by no means immune. While the greater part of this book will be found to apply to women in particular, there is a special section for men.

CHAPTER ONE

Cystitis – the Most Common Causes

To begin, it is useful to have an idea of the different types of cystitis there are. In order to plan a treatment the cause must be determined, so have a look through the following paragraphs to see which is most likely to apply to you. Then refer to the Appendix for the dietary tables.

UTERUS OUT OF POSITION

As will be seen from Figure 1, the uterus can tilt over the bladder and press down on it, causing it to fold over at the bottom, or at least to have a pocket of urine which cannot fall out when the valve opens to empty the bladder. This urine becomes stale and a breeding ground for infection, which quickly irritates the bladder lining and causes pain and all the classic symptoms. Copious drinking will tend to dilute the urine and therefore the infection, but, of course, is no cure and in any event results in even more frequency. Antibiotics may kill the

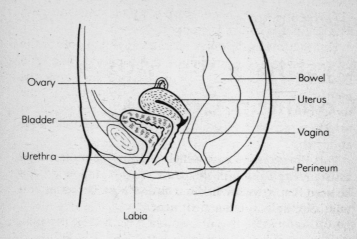

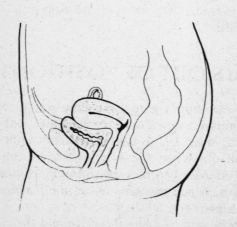

Figure 1. (a) Bladder and uterus in normal position. (b) Anteverted uterus causing compression of the bladder.

infection, but it may often return as a more resistant strain as soon as the course is stopped.

This type of cystitis often becomes apparent only as the uterus becomes heavy coming up to period time, and heals as the weight of the uterus is reduced by the menstrual flow. However, if severe, it may continue throughout the cycle, particularly if the uterus is subject to other pressures, such as fibroids or post-operative adhesions.

This situation is a case which often needs professional assistance to deal with the cause, but the following can be used first, which will often clear the milder cases and will back up any other treatment.

Treatment

EXERCISE
The exercise (a) described on page 63 is most important for this condition and should be carried out religiously morning and evening and after any period of prolonged standing.

DIET
The Cleansing Diet on page 49 is important to help the tissues to heal quickly once the bladder returns to its normal shape.

HERBS
Herbal treatments are often effective in helping quick tissue recovery. Parsley Piert (obtainable in tablet form) is a safe and convenient home remedy.

HYDROTHERAPY
Hydrotherapy is a most effective home treatment to increase blood circulation and drainage in the bladder area and tone the supporting muscles and ligaments. At its simplest, spray your middle with alternate hot and cold water, morning and night, about six fifteen-second applications of each, starting with hot and finishing with cold. *Always* splash or spray cold water around the feet, legs and lower abdomen after a hot bath.

For the more stubborn condition, Sitz baths should be used. Place two large, deep plastic basins in the bath. Fill one with hot water (as hot as you can stand) and the other with cold (even slightly iced) water. Sit in the hot with feet in the cold for about a half to one minute, then reverse the procedure and sit in the cold. Three or four cycles will get a vigorous rush of blood circulating through the lower body, giving the damaged tissues good nourishment and drainage for the quick renewal.

REFLEXOLOGY
The Foot Reflex Points for the bladder will be very tender and easily found by gentle probing in the area (see page 35). Fingertips or knuckle massage, using a slight

clockwise kneading motion will gradually reduce the pain and should be repeated on alternate days until all pain has gone. Stop the massage for any one day as soon as the foot begins to sweat.

There are various other specialist treatments, any one of which might be appropriate for you, as discussed on pages 27–37.

BLADDER OUT OF POSITION

Excessive strain on the lower abdomen through awkward lifting etc., especially when combined with a heavy and protruding abdomen, can result in prolapse of the bladder. The supporting tissues fail to hold it in position and it slumps downward, causing much the same symptoms as in the last section (Uterus Out of Position) except that there is less involvement of the menstrual cycle. Normally there would be a dragging or bearing down sensation and occasionally the bladder may even become visible through its orifice, though this is an extreme condition requiring surgical treatment.

Treatment

EXERCISE
The exercise (a) described on page 63 morning and evening and after prolonged standing. A general physical fitness and if necessary weight reduction programme.

Leg raising exercises to tone the abdominal wall – (b) on page 64.

DIET
The Cleansing Diet on page 49 followed after 7-10 days by the Yang diet for tissue strengthening (page 50).

HERBS
Tissue toning and constricting herbs supplied by a Medical Herbalist will be most useful.

HYDROTHERAPY
As detailed in the previous section, hydrotherapy will increase the tone and circulation of the bladder and its attachments, helping it regain the strength to hold itself in position. The Sitz baths are especially recommended.

REFLEXOLOGY
The Foot Reflex Points (see Figure 3 on page 35) should be massaged with quick vigorous movements until the feet start to sweat. This will probably only take a minute or so on the first day but will take longer on subsequent days.

ACUPUNCTURE
Acupuncture and moxabustion (an associated treatment) are invaluable in this condition and should dramatically shorten the healing time.

INFECTION OF THE BLADDER

The bladder may become infected either downwards from the kidneys or upwards from the urethra in addition to the conditions previously described where infection is generated within the bladder itself. If the source comes down from the kidneys it is likely to be much more painful in that area and treatment would be directed at the kidneys, not the bladder.

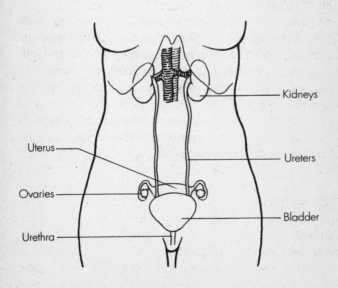

Figure 2. Front view of the urinary system.

More common, however, is infection caused by 'bugs' invading the urethra from the vaginal or penis area. They breed under bad hygienic conditions, ideal living conditions being found under the male foreskin and in the warm, moist vagina. Regular washing and douching is important for all, especially before and after intercourse.

Non-Specific Urethritis (NSU) is a very common condition nowadays, particularly in women who have had a confinement or other treatment in hospital, where their genito-urinary system is exposed to hardy, drug-resistant strains of infective organisms. The other main method of transmission is sexual intercourse.

Symptoms of infection are usually frequency with burning pain on passing water, also persistent pain or ache in the lower abdomen. There may be difficulty in passing water, and it may come in small amounts.

Antibiotic treatments may suppress the symptoms somewhat but do not often clear the condition completely. If you have persistent distressing symptoms see your doctor, who will probably wish to have a urine culture prepared and analysed.

Treatment

HYGIENE
Obviously, scrupulous cleanliness. Also, good ventilation to prevent breeding of anaerobic bacteria (which are killed by contact with the air). As with all cystitis, nylon tights and pants should be avoided. Clothing in the area should be loose fitting and changed regularly.

If possible, intercourse should be avoided – to avoid spreading the infection or being re-infected. If you do have intercourse, pass as much urine as possible soon after, to flush any foreign bodies away from the urethra.

HERBS

Internal bathing with 1 to 10 solution of Tincture of Calendula (obtainable from Herbalists and good Health Stores) night and morning will reduce inflammation and help clear infection.

Application of a mixture of vitamin E and calendula cream, obtainable from health stores, will be most helpful in reducing local surface irritation, should this be present.

DIET

A complete fast may be necessary, preceded by the Cleansing Diet (see page 49).

STRESS

A surprising amount of cystitis is due to emotional stress of one sort or another. It is often difficult to identify the cause for oneself, because almost by definition there has been a suppression of recognition of the cause at a conscious level, and the tension is pushed, unrecognized, down into the physical body.

Of course, very many symptoms are produced in this way. Depending on the basic emotion being suppressed, different parts of the body will be affected. For instance, suppressed aggression will cause frozen shoulders; a desire to run away, hip and leg problems; and fear, water difficulties.

While a severe fright is widely known to cause wetting of the pants in some people, a long-standing or recurring background fear may give quite severe cystitis symptoms, which can mimic many of the other causes mentioned in this chapter.

A case history may be useful to illustrate this. Mrs V, who had never had any history of bladder problems, had a lot of difficulty persuading her husband to give their daughter the kind of wedding she considered appropriate. The husband became very rebellious and even on the day of the ceremony threatened to disrupt it. At the reception, Mrs V suddenly contracted violent cystitis and was plagued with it for the next twelve years, until on the day her husband died she suddenly found herself free of it. In the years since, she has not had a trace of it.

The trouble with this condition is that most of us have to cope with various stresses and it is very easy to say 'Oh, it's all in the mind – just worry', and miss the true origin completely. If you have carefully read the descriptions of all the other types, and nothing quite fits your problem, *then* have a good think about what was happening in your life when you had your first attack.

Treatment

DIET

Remember, the basic emotion involved is *fear* – of a person, sex, thing or situation. You must build up your resistance to fear, by eating more Yang, acid-producing foods, nourishing your 'water' energy by keeping away from cold conditions and foods and getting plenty of rest.

BACH FLOWER REMEDIES

The Bach remedies *Mimulus* (for fear of a known origin) and *Aspen* (fear of unknown origin), obtainable from homoeopathic pharmacies, will be most helpful.

ACUPUNCTURE

Acupuncture is a particularly good way of building up the deficient water energy, and is highly recommended as a next step should self-treatment be insufficient.

EXCESSIVE ACIDITY/ALKALINITY

Nature normally maintains a neutral balance between acidity and alkalinity of urine in the bladder at a figure of about pH 6.8. Should it become more alkaline the pH will rise to perhaps 7.2, and if acid (more common) will drop to perhaps 5.6. Litmus-based test-sticks may be bought from a chemist which will tell you whether the urine has gone one way or the other. Do not go on the results of one test only, however, as the value may reflect your last meal! Take a mid-stream sample first thing in the morning, then compare it with further samples taken later in the day.

Deviation from neutral pH will cause a burning irritation of the sensitive membranes of the urethra, resulting in a fairly continuous dull burning pain which is likely to worsen during and just after passing water. Of course, the more irritated the membranes become, the more the bladder is stimulated to empty and so there is often associated frequency.

This condition may often be present in conjunction with other factors, so it is wise to check for it in all cases of bladder irritation. In addition to the annoying local symptoms, long-standing acidity can cause precipitation of calcium out of the urine in the kidneys to form uric acid calculi or stones. Correction of the pH over a period of time will encourage absorption of these stones back into the urine for painless clearance.

Treatment

DIET

Study of the diets listed towards the end of this book will clearly show which foods produce acid and alkaline reactions in the urine. It is normally quite easy to control the balance by careful eating, but in exceptional cases a proprietary remedy may be required, such as Uralyt U (obtainable only through a naturopathic practitioner).

Provided the pH stays within the range 6.6 to 7.0 there will be no irritation from this source. During a fast, of course, the reading will become quite high and should be disregarded.

Bacterial pathogens love an acid environment, so the chances of infection will be kept to a minimum by careful dietary control. In emergency, a level teaspoonful of bicarbonate of soda dissolved in half a pint (275ml) of water and taken every hour for three hours will usually reduce a severe attack of cystitis.

CYSTITIS IN MEN

As mentioned earlier, cystitis is normally thought of as a female complaint, but is no less distressing when it occurs in the male. The most common form of urinary disturbance in the man is of course due to prostate gland enlargement, which causes restriction of the urethra and brings about painful water retention problems. This does not properly come under the heading of cystitis, so we shall concentrate on the other main cause of irritation – infection.

Infection can range from gonorrhoea – passing razor blades is the best description I have heard of its early symptoms – through NSU to very minor bacterial cultures. If there is or has recently been an external lesion on the genitals it could indicate some form of venereal infection and you should see your doctor immediately. A straightforward irritation/frequency should be tackled in the same way as described in the preceding sections 'Infection of the Bladder' and 'Excessive Acidity/Alkalinity'. In the event of irritation occurring only following ejaculation, medical or homoeopathic treatment may be required.

CYSTITIS FOLLOWING INTERCOURSE

A large proportion of cystitis sufferers find that their complaint relates largely, if not entirely, to the act of sexual intercourse. Many marriages come under great strain and indeed breakdown because of the disastrous consequences of physical union. Often within minutes of making love, the vaginal and bladder area becomes painful, spreading across the whole lower abdomen to the low back. Within two to three hours blood appears in the urine, which is only passed with excruciating pain and often uncontrollably.

The factors which may be involved here are:

Bruising Leading to Infection

This occurs particularly after prolonged and vigorous activity. It may also occur if the female vaginal secretions are inadequate to provide proper lubrication or the internal organs are out of position or full – a laden bowel or bladder will cause more pressure around the sexual area.

Direct Infection

The bacteria E Coli, which lives normally and happily in the bowel, tends to cross the perineum (the small piece of skin between the anus and vagina) very easily if hygiene is less than scrupulous and is virtually pumped into the vagina and urethra by sexual activity. It breeds in warmth and damp, and within minutes just a few bacteria can form a sizeable culture in the urethral area.

The underside of the male foreskin is again an ideal area for bacteria, so they are deposited neatly into the receptive vagina if the area is not kept clean.

Why cystitis sufferers are more susceptible in general to these minor traumas of tissue has not yet been satisfactorily explained. For some reason, the tissues more readily support bacterial migration and multiplication than usual – after all, everyone carries multitudes of bacteria around with them. However, it is known that these bacteria thrive in an acid environment so we must of course increase the alkalinity of the tissues.

Treatment

DIET
As a first step, the well-known routine of a teaspoonful of bicarbonate of soda with half a pint (275ml) of water or cordial will immediately ensure that the descending urine becomes more alkaline, and this should be followed up with the alkaline-producing diet on page 56.

To establish when your pH is under control, obtain a jar of Litmus-based test-sticks from your chemist. When dipped in a urine sample they will show the pH on a colour chart. This should be kept at between 6.8 and 7.0. Most cystitis sufferers who have come to my surgery have had a pH of around 5.8 to 6.0 and of course this reflects not only acidity of the urine but also of the tissues, which encourage the travel of bacteria from one point to another.

A PREVENTIVE ROUTINE

A very simple and often effective step is to make sure you pass water after intercourse – preferably within a few minutes. This flushes out the urethra, washing away any bacteria that are trying to climb up the urethra towards the bladder. Then shower vigorously and thoroughly in and around the vaginal area with cold water, and finish by bathing the urethral area with tincture of calendula or witch hazel on cotton wool.

HOMOEOPATHY

An effective homoeopathic remedy for cystitis following intercourse is *Staphisagria*, taken orally in a potency of about 12x.

ALLERGIES

As the number and complexity of chemical substances in modern life increases, more and more people are starting to suffer allergic reactions. These can affect the bladder just as easily as the lungs, sinuses or skin. In particular, vaginal deodorants, talcum powders and scented soaps and bath oils should be avoided. Often, even apparently simple substances will contain all sorts of complex chemical additives. If in doubt, stick to 'Simple Soap' and water.

Foodstuffs may well cause cystitis – and not just

chemically adulterated ones! Raw carrots and beetroot can have an intensely irritating effect on the bladder and urethra, even in quite small quantities, in susceptible people. Heavily chlorinated water can be responsible, which would of course aggravate an attack should you follow the usual routine and flush the system with lots of it!

Alcohol is most undesirable for cystitis sufferers as it raises the urinary acidity and causes dehydration. In addition to this general problem, some people may find that a particular drink, such as red wine or perhaps sherry, causes a more severe reaction. These should obviously be avoided. If you do wish to drink, have a 'long one' – beer is best – or a long mixed drink, preferably not containing a highly aromatic alcohol such as brandy or whisky. If you know you are going to drink, have a soft (non-citrus) half-pint before and after.

Treatment

DIET

Should you suspect a dietary allergy, first try changing to the diet on page 54. If this does not work, check your pulse rate before, and half-an-hour after, eating every meal, and write it down along with the contents of the meal. An allergic reaction will normally reveal itself by an abnormal change of pulse rate following the meal. Then you must try each ingredient of the meal separately until the allergen has been isolated.

Practitioners of Applied Kinesiology, Clinical Kinesiology and EAV (Electro-Acupuncture according to

Voll) have specific diagnostic methods for determining allergies and effective treatments for eliminating them. In particular, any member of the world-wide International College of Applied Kinesiology will be specifically trained in treatment of allergies.

AVOID CHEMICALS

Hexachlorophene has fortunately now been banned from inclusion in toothpaste and children's toiletries, but is frequently used in medicated shampoos, soaps and powders. Hexachlorophene is really bad news for cystitis sufferers and must be carefully avoided. Do not have it in the house at all!

CHAPTER TWO

Alternative Approaches to Treatment

Cystitis is at best embarrassing and uncomfortable and at worst dangerous. As we have seen from the last chapter, it can arise from quite complex causes. Unfortunately, although it occurs in acute bursts, it is usually a deeply entrenched chronic condition which surfaces in the presence of an irritant. For this reason, some people have to accept that management of their condition is all they can achieve – the tissues may have become permanently damaged and prevent a complete cure.

If you have had recurring bladder trouble for some time, the chances are you have had at least one bladder cystoscopy, and possibly an IVP (intravenous pyelogram – kidney x-ray), loads of antibiotics and still get cystitis, with the possible added bonus of thrush. Cystitis is very resistant to symptomatic treatment, such as painkillers and antibiotics.

There are other effective approaches and we shall now have a brief look at them. As will be seen in the table in the Appendix, different therapies may be preferable in particular cases.

NATURE CURE

The naturopath is concerned with simple, direct approaches to improving the health of the whole body. The core of naturopathic treatment is dietary management, with which this book is primarily concerned. This is used in conjunction with hydrotherapy (see the methods described on page 12) to encourage blood-flow and drainage through the abdominal organs. This therapy, while deceptively simple, will prove to be your most effective tool, and it is free! However, should you follow all the advice in this book and still not fully recover, a naturopath may be able to give you more detailed treatment, 'made-to-measure'.

OSTEOPATHY

Should the problem be due to malpositioning of any of the internal organs, or from irritation of the nervous system, osteopathy will be required. A good osteopath works just as much with the soft tissues as with bones, and that includes the internal organs. It is usually a simple matter to replace an anteverted uterus manually – this is done during an internal examination, so be prepared! Some osteopaths tend to specialize in gynaecological problems and they will be particularly helpful.

In general, the theory behind osteopathy is that the body tissues need a strong, unimpaired supply of nervous signals, blood and lymph. Any obstructions to these are removed by resolving congestion and tension of soft tissue and mobilizing restricted joints. Posture is corrected where this is a problem – many people almost *give* themselves abdominal problems by allowing the pelvis to tilt forward, throwing the tummy forward over the bladder. Have a look at your profile in the mirror!

ACUPUNCTURE

You will have noticed a few rather peculiar statements in the last chapter referring to Yin, Yang, 'energy' etc. This is because I find the Oriental concept of health and disease extremely useful in practice. Using it, one can gain an overall picture of the strengths and weaknesses of a person, and by balancing these, reduce the tendency to disease.

If the body energy and vitality is sufficiently raised, all the weak tissues will be repaired and renewed – nature always works towards health. Acupuncture gives it a hefty punch in the right direction, in a more specific and accurate way than Nature Cure. Although both systems help nature to cure, acupuncture diagnosis is so sophisticated and accurate that, used correctly, almost instant improvement can be expected.

Like all natural medicines, of course, it works best with active, functional tissue – scar tissue or other pathological degenerations which involve changes of tissue structure tend to be more permanent. Even so, by improving the function of tissue surrounding the degenerated area much improvement can be felt. For instance, deep abdominal adhesions due to post-operative scarring respond excellently – and almost instantly – to local acupuncture needles, especially when combined with laser and/or magnet treatment.

Like Nature Cure, acupuncture pays a lot of attention to diet. Foods are divided into those which are more Yin or more Yang, and those which might introduce 'external evils' such as chill into the body. While a general picture of Yin and Yang foods is given on page 51, you should really see an acupuncturist to have a diet based on his observation of your individual Yin/Yang balance.

HERBALISM

Herbalism can be complementary to acupuncture, but it is difficult to have it prescribed in the Oriental manner in the West i.e. hot herbs for cold conditions, drying herbs for wet conditions etc. Medical herbalism as practised in Britain, while using a different basis for prescription (more like orthodox medicine in that concoctions are made up mainly on a study of symptomatology), is a very effective solution to many health problems. For many hundreds of years the efficacy of various plants has been recognized; indeed, some plants, such as pilewort, are named after their medicinal uses.

JUNIPER BERRIES
Before consulting a herbalist, you might like to try having an infusion of juniper berries every morning and evening for a week or so, in addition to the other procedures

described elsewhere. This fruit is particularly good for toning the kidneys, but is also effective in the acute stage of cystitis.

ASPARAGUS

Asparagus is a very good general conditioner for all bladder and kidney troubles. Preferably use the fresh, juicy, raw shoots which top this attractive ferny plant in the spring. If you do not have any in the garden buy it at good greengrocers, or even use the canned asparagus tips, which still contain enough asparagin (its specific remedial component) to be effective. The ferny leaves can also be made up as a tea. Put a large cupful of the leaves in a stainless steel or enamel pot, add two cupfuls of water, and heat until almost, but not quite, boiling. Allow to cool, keeping the lid on the pot, leave overnight and decant, complete with leaves, into a jar which can be covered with muslin. Two dessertspoonfuls twice a day should be drunk, hot or cold, using a tea-strainer to collect stray leaves.

HORSETAIL

Horsetail (*Equisetum arvense*) is used for all inflammatory troubles of the uterus, vagina and bladder. Allow the whole plant (usually found on waste ground and in ditches) to dry, break it up and brew one dessertspoonful in one and a half pints (850ml) of water as above. Take two dessertspoonsful morning and night. Use it as a douche as well – pulp the herb, dissolve a handful in a pint (575ml) of warm vinegar, and dilute with a pint (575ml) of water.

HYDRANGEA

Hydrangea, that ubiquitous flowering shrub found in most British gardens, is another useful medicament for kidney and bladder inflammation. Prepare a brew of the chopped leaves as described for asparagus; take two dessertspoonsful morning and night.

HOMOEOPATHY

Since its discovery by Samuel Hahnemann in the late eighteenth century, homoeopathy has had a large and devoted following. It is based on the idea of like curing like, so that if you have cystitis you take a very diluted form of a substance which, when taken in a more normal dose, would actually *produce* cystitis. The process of dilution is known as 'potentization', and the higher the potency, or dilution, the deeper acting the remedy. For the acute physical symptoms of cystitis a low potency of, say, 6x will work well, but for the more subtle psycho-emotional factors which may lie behind it, a much higher potency – even up to a one in six million dilution – may be needed.

While many people prescribe their own remedies (which are easily obtainable from homoeopathic pharmacies in many cities) from the indications given in repertories and Materia Medicas, it should be realized that effective prescription is a very highly skilled technique which it takes much study and years of experience to learn. The few remedies mentioned elsewhere may be tried first, especially if you have no homoeopath near you, but should they not have the desired effect within a few weeks, a detailed consultation with a homoeopath may be the right key for your particular lock. For instance, different remedies are prescribed for each of the following conditions, and these should be backed up by other constitutional remedies. One may develop cystitis:

- after intercourse
- before period
- during period
- with constipation
- with evacuation
- with stress
- with excitement
- with cold weather
- at night
- with drinking particular fluids
- with spasmodic sphincter contraction with straining

Each condition indicates the use of different remedies.

ALLOPATHY (ORTHODOX MEDICINE)

Modern medicine is very good at telling you what bacteria has infected your bladder, whether it has reached the kidneys, whether there is any visible scarring or polyp (by cystoscopy) or whether there is any congenital abnormality or renal calculus which might occasion recurring infection (usually by x-ray using an intravenous dye). Some conditions thus diagnosed may respond to surgery, but these belong to a small minority of cystitis sufferers.

Functional treatment tends to be with antibiotics and chemicals. Nitrofurantoin is one of the most common chemicals and it can create a hostile environment for bacterial infection. Various antibiotics are prescribed – tetracyclines, penicillin, ampicillin, and the sulphonamides being the most common. It has been my experience, however, that while these substances often bring about immediate improvement, some bugs usually survive and start a drug-resistant strain, so that another, stronger drug with more side-effects has to be used next time.

One of the common results of taking antibiotics is thrush, a fungus condition of the vagina. Not only does the antibiotic kill the bad germs, it also kills the good ones which keep such conditions at bay. A subsequent fungicide then needs to be prescribed, which in turn runs the risk of having to be varied should another attack occur.

REFLEXOLOGY

Foot Reflex Therapy is a very old technique originating in the Far East, but developed and publicized mainly by Eunice Ingham in the USA. It is a marvellous technique for both diagnosis and treatment at home. Books and charts relating to it can be obtained through good libraries and bookshops.

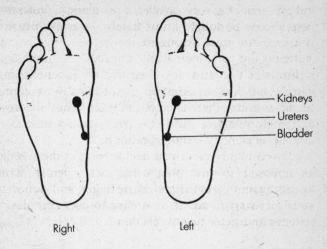

Figure 3. Foot reflexes of kidneys, ureters and bladder.

The feet contain thousands of nerve endings which connect with other parts of the body through reflex arcs in the central nervous system. When an organ becomes distressed, the appropriate area of the feet also becomes tender, even swollen in more acute cases. Massage of these tender areas sends a nervous stimulus to the organ and assists healing.

From a diagnostic point of view alone reflexology can be of great assistance in determining just where the cystitis is active. As shown in Figure 3, the positions of the bladder, ureter and kidneys are quite precise. If the inflammation has gone half-way up the ureter on the left, this can be easily established from the feet. Should the kidney areas be very swollen and tender, professional help should be sought immediately – it is not worth the risk trying to treat it yourself.

There are an increasing number of professional reflexologists around, and their treatment benefits many cystitis sufferers. In addition to specifically treating the bladder and other affected reflexes, this therapy is extremely relaxing and helps considerably in resolving any stress element in the condition.

A word of advice. If you decide to treat these reflexes as opposed to just diagnosing, start gently with a kneading motion of the pad of the finger, and stop should your feet start to sweat. It is easy to over-stimulate the reflexes and get a heavy reaction!

The Ear

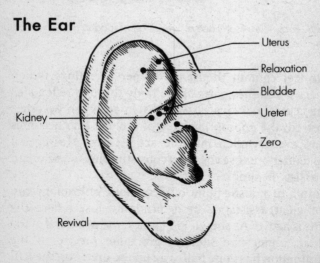

Figure 4. Treatment points in the ear.

The ears, like the feet, have reflex points that correspond to the organs of the body. These points are especially good for controlling an acute condition.

Use a probe such as an old ball-point pen or a matchstick, taking care not to let it actually enter the ear, to gently palpate the relevant areas. The areas needing treatment will be exquisitely tender. Knead the painful points gently with the instrument, or even your finger-nail, for a couple of minutes or so, until the point becomes less painful. Repeat a few hours later.

CHAPTER THREE

The Importance
of Diet

All our organs depend for their health on balanced
nutrition and drainage. Each individual cell is nourished
by food-rich fluid and its waste material is continually
washed away. If the food borne in this fluid is lacking in
something or has too much congestive material, the
delicate exchange is upset and the cells become anoxic
(lacking in oxygen), slow to reproduce and prone to
damage from infection. They would then be unable to
cope adequately with fluctuating environmental
conditions – for instance, too much acidity, dryness, chill
or bruising. So the body loses its resilience and becomes
prone to all sorts of ailments, cystitis included.

One can look at nutrition in various ways. The
advertisements tell us we should buy item A because it
is cheap, item B because it is quick to prepare, item C
because it keeps well, item D because it has added
vitamins and minerals, and item E because it is
fashionable. Some even persuade us to buy things
because they are expensive! Health magazines and books
offer all sorts of permutations of 'natural' foods, often

augmented by expensive supplements. And, of course, most of us tend to eat what happens to be around at the time.

There is no easy answer to dietary problems, because we are all different. The old saying 'One man's meat is another man's poison' is very true. Depending on our constitution, we may need lots of protein, or lots of fruit (seldom both). The more sensitive person will probably have quite distinct messages from the digestive system, and may well instinctively eat the right things. Many of us, unfortunately, have had our palate dulled by years of ill-advised eating and do not pick up the messages until we are actually ill. Even then, it tends to be some 'bug', not the food, that is assumed to have caused the trouble.

You would not try to run your car on paraffin but so many expect their bodies to function on much worse! Try reading the list of ingredients on a soup packet, a cola bottle or a pre-mixed dessert. If there is anything of nutritional value there, it must surely be an accident! But even if you are already food-conscious, it is easy to eat an imbalance of the best organically grown foods and still become ill. For instance, the odd cystitis sufferer will have immediate relief if they stop eating all those raw carrots. More commonly, however, an over-acid blood supply is the predisposing factor, and the only logical long-term control of this is through careful eating habits.

Green vegetables, with their high calcium to phosphorus ratio, control harmful acids most effectively. For instance, the calcium to phosphorus ratio in lettuce is 1 to 0.6, while in beef it is about 1 to 1.3.

ACID/ALKALINE BALANCE

The importance of a good acid/alkali (base) equilibrium could hardly be put more clearly than by Alexander Nelson in his book *Medical Botany*.

> Minerals are of great importance because they enter into the components of tissue elements or facilitate functions, but their service does not end there. Many are of use in maintaining osmotic equilibria within and between tissues. Again, the acid/base equilibrium within the body is of first-class importance and is affected by the diet. The body excretes excess of either anions or cations, but ingestion of a diet supplying over-much of either places an extra strain on the mechanisms of excretion. For example, it had long been known that foodstuffs like meat, eggs, and cereals have an 'acid ash', fruits and vegetables an 'anti-acid ash'. In sickness, acidosis occurs oftener and is to be feared more than alkalosis. For these and other reasons, from amongst plant foodstuffs, it is advisable to incorporate fruits and vegetables in a diet rather than excess cereals.

While all the dietary minerals are of great importance, some can be almost taken for granted provided a reasonably mixed food intake from varied areas is consumed. One of the most well-known cases of deficiency has been iodine, which before the addition of this mineral to household salt led to goitre – 'Derbyshire Neck' because of the lack of iodine in local Derbyshire produce. However, a subtle but continued relative imbalance of minerals is often present in the modern 'civilized' diet, due to the predilection for processed foods.

CALCIUM/PHOSPHORUS

Calcium is a most important mineral, not only for bones and teeth but in the blood and all cellular structures. It can only be made available to the body in the presence of phosphorus in the ratio of approximately 1 to 1. There are various factors which can upset the proper absorption and use of calcium, one of the most important of which is phytin. This substance is found in plants in various forms. The B vitamin inositol is one, it also combines as an acid ester with various minerals to form calcium phytate, magnesium phytate etc. If hydrolyzed, however, these substances will block the mineral uptake. For example, if phytin is present and is hydrolyzed (as happens in the leavening of bread and food processing) phosphoric acid is released which reacts with dietary calcium and forms insoluble calcium phosphate which cannot be absorbed. A diet high in phytin content will therefore severely interfere with calcium, and also, in the same way, magnesium and iron.

Most leaf vegetables, swede and turnip, are free from phytin. Carrots and parsnips have quite a lot, and the cereals contain a high quantity. Pulses have a high phytin content. The greener the leaf, the more absorbable calcium, with its attendant phosphorus, it is likely to contain. The outer leaves of cabbage, for instance, and water-cress are very rich in calcium. Spinach has lots too, but it is undesirable in quantity because of its high oxalate content.

The modern practice of adding phosphate fertilizers to the soil tends to markedly reduce the level of calcium in all plants, and can be dangerous in some cases – spinach grown in this way has been found to have caused the death of infants.

Both calcium and phosphorus depend for their uptake, in both plant and man, on magnesium. This metal is found in all the body tissues. The primary source is again the dark green vegetables as it is a component of the chlorophyll molecule which gives the plant its green colour. Almonds and brazil nuts also contain significant amounts of magnesium.

Balanced calcium/magnesium tablets are readily available from health food shops, should you find difficulty in obtaining enough from fresh organic vegetables.

IRON

Iron is, of course, vital to health, as anyone who suffers from anaemia knows only too well. Without it the haemoglobin level of the blood drops, and oxygen cannot be carried adequately by the blood, leading to deterioration of the cell tone and vulnerability to infection and disease.

Normally there is no deficiency of iron in a varied diet, but again modern farming methods prejudice our iron intake, as nitrogenous fertilizers lower the iron content of crops by about a third. This figure can be further reduced by lack of organic matter being returned to the soil, because it is this which reduces iron to a soluble form for uptake by the plant. The moral is, therefore, grow your own food where possible, using compost as fertilizer. Failing that, take a multi-mineral supplement.

SODIUM/POTASSIUM BALANCE

This is critical to nerve and cell functioning in the body. Normally we all get quite sufficient amounts of both minerals in our diet, but in recurring cystitis there may well be a shortage of potassium in conjunction with acidosis. Again, vegetables are a primary source of potassium. Sodium i.e. sodium chloride – common salt – should be used sparingly as over-use upsets the balance between the two minerals and attracts water.

The balance between internal and external fluids at a cellular level is determined largely by the sodium/potassium levels. There is a predominance of potassium (as phosphate and bicarbonate compounds) in the interstitial fluid. There is a dynamic tension between these groups which results in good transport of nutrients and waste across the cell boundaries. Should there be a significant imbalance between the concentrations of the two, the tissues will be too dry or too wet, and health will decline. If both are inadequate there will be slow, lazy metabolism causing sluggishness and susceptibility to infection.

Virtually everything we eat contains both sodium and

potassium. The acid reaction foods are particularly high in sodium; the alkaline reaction food contain a higher predominance of potassium. In the acidic condition which breeds cystitis, therefore, we need to concentrate on getting plenty of potassium-rich foods, which have a cleansing and soothing effect.

All foods have more potassium than sodium, but the ratio varies enormously. For health, we should have an average of somewhere around 100 parts of potassium to one of sodium. Listed below are some foods with their potassium/sodium ratio.

Cherries	280:1
Bananas	400:1
Pears	180:1
Oats	170:1
Potatoes	40:1
Rice	100:1
Oranges	125:1

SULPHUR

Again this mineral is essential to health, but if taken in excess leads to an acid ash, which is what we must avoid. The main source of sulphur is probably sulphur dioxide which is used as a preservative in dried fruits and fruit juices. Sun-dried fruits are hard to find, but if you are fond of dried fruits they are worth the effort.

Homoeopathic *Sulphur* 6x or 10x is a good 'spring

cleaning' remedy and helps clear excess sulphur from the body.

VITAMINS

Vitamins are substances which act as catalysts to produce necessary metabolic functions within the body. It is unusual in the west to see clinical vitamin deficiencies, as even processed and denatured foods often have vitamins – albeit synthetic – added to comply with food regulations. There are many detailed sources of information on vitamins and their importance, but all the diets shown in the following chapter should have more than sufficient for health. Where a deficiency has developed, perhaps through incorrect absorption or excessive stress, a supplement may be indicated, and this is normally prescribed on the basis of deficiency symptoms. For instance, dry, irritated vaginal tissues will often respond to vitamin A (found in fish liver oil), coated tongue to the B complex, sore gums to vitamin C, anoxia (lack of oxygen in the tissues leading to bad circulation and drainage) to vitamin E.

An important cause of vitamin deficiency is incorrect food preparation. Over-cooking, peeling and shredding of fruits and vegetables will almost totally lose their water-soluble vitamin content, especially vitamin C (the B complex is the other main water-soluble group). Fat-soluble vitamins – A, D, E and K – will be lost through frying etc. Canning causes a very high level of vitamin destruction. For instance, the carotene content of carrots drops from 19.90 to 12.80, thiamin from 0.07 to 0.04 and niacin from 0.56 to 0.36. Other convenience foods fare even worse; dried mashed potato, for example, loses 81 per cent of its vitamin C, which is one of the potato's most important ingredients.

FOOD PREPARATION

The golden rule is keep it simple. Why laboriously peel and dice carrots when a good scrub will do? Nature has protected the rich abundance of nutrients with a thin, tasteless skin, why throw it away? If you want them diced, do it just before serving. Why boil vegetables at all? Steaming keeps all the flavour in, keeps them crisper and much more nutritious. What about a delicious pre-dinner cocktail – the vegetable water with perhaps a dash of yeast extract will be better for you than any tonic you buy in the chemist shop!

We have talked a lot about vegetables because they are so important in a cystitis diet, but obviously care should be taken with other foods too. If you are having meat, try to avoid 'factory farm' products, which are reared on concentrates and are usually stuffed full of antibiotics, and often hormones. Proprietary foods such as fish fingers, frozen pizzas, beefburgers etc., will usually contain all sorts of chemical additives, and should be avoided for this reason, quite apart from their dubious food value. If frying or sautéing, use a good quality sunflower or safflower oil and do not do it often. Stir-frying with garlic and ginger preserves the goodness of the oil and the food.

Perhaps the most important part of food preparation is to prepare yourself to eat it. If you have a good supply of saliva, teeth which will masticate the food properly, and a happy, relaxed stomach able to supply the right gastric juices for the food coming down, you will be able to get away with all sorts of dietary indiscretions. The best food in the world will be harmful to you if you snatch it in a sandwich while upset and in a hurry. Think for a moment of what you are going to eat, sit down calmly and enjoy it. Prepared with love, the foods given in this book will taste superb to a receptive palate.

Table 1. Potential Acidity of Acid-ash Foods

Acid-ash Foods	Potential Acidity (ml normal acid per 100 grams)
Oatmeal	12
Rice	9
Wheat (entire)	12
Wheat flour	9
White bread	6
Grilled beefsteak	23
Roast chicken	25
Leg of mutton	22.5
Roast pork	28.6

Table 2. Potential Alkalinity of Alkaline-ash Foods

Alkaline-ash Foods	Potential Alkalinity (ml normal alkali per 100 grams)
Apples	3
Bananas	8
Dried Beans	10
Fresh Beans	5
Fresh Beet	10
Carrots	14
Dates	9
Lemon	4
Olives	45
Onions	1
Orange	5
Pears	4
Potatoes	9
Radishes	5
Swedes	8
Tomatoes	5
Turnips	11
Water Melon	4

(Source: *Chemistry of Food & Nutrition* by H. C. Sherman, McMillan.)

CHAPTER FOUR

Diets and Recipes

CLEANSING DIET

For a minimum of 3 days, maximum 7 days.

Suggested Menu

BREAKFAST
¼ lb (100g) grapes
Apple or grape juice

MID-MORNING
Cup of lemon tea

LUNCH
Mixed fruit salad, with some mixed nuts
'Live' yogurt

MID-AFTERNOON
Cup of lemon tea

EVENING MEAL

Mixed salad without cheese, meat, fish or mayonnaise.
A little apple cider vinegar and sunflower oil can be used
for dressing.
Non-citrus fruit, fruit juice.

ON RETIRING

A cup of peppermint or chamomile tea.

As an aid to elimination, have an Epsom Salts bath on
alternate nights just before retiring. Put one to one and a
half pounds (675g) of Epsom Salts in a hot bath, and soak
in it for twenty minutes, then dry quickly and go straight
to bed. This will induce profuse sweating which will help
the general body elimination. DO NOT have an Epsom
Salts bath during an actual attack of cystitis, however.

YANG DIET

This diet, as explained on page 19, is normally for use
where the cystitis is due to emotional causes, especially
that of fear. The person needing this diet will be easily
depressed, and their body will probably be watery and
overweight. It contains more acid foods than would
normally be desirable, but nothing extreme.

In Oriental medicine, the Yang concept is of a dry,
dense, concentrated food containing more sodium than
potassium. It is the stimulating, body building polarity as
opposed to the cleansing, sedating effect of the more
watery Yin foods.

The system of Macrobiotics is based on the achievement of an ideal Yin/Yang balance in all food intake, and while I think the general concept is a good one, most of the popular publications on the subject tend to suggest a regime which leads to severe deficiency of vitamin C and, in some cases, protein. In the final analysis, your body will tell you what it needs if you listen to it. This diet may be applicable to you for a few weeks, or even months, but it should be gradually enlarged to cover more Yin (fruit and vegetables) foods as your appetite demands them. An advantage of this macrobiotic approach is that it nourishes the psyche and increases self-perception.

Suggested Menu

BREAKFAST
Unsweetened muesli cereal base with mixed dried fruits, moistened with water or natural yogurt.
One cup Mu tea (obtainable from health stores and grain shops).

LUNCH
Brown rice and cooked (preferably sautéd) mixed seasonal vegetables,
or rice balls,
or tempura with rice (see recipes below).
Miso stew

EVENING MEAL
Brown rice with sautéd seasonal vegetables and/or bean stew or tempura or seaweed.

Or buckwheat, millet or wholewheat soaked, boiled and dressed with soy sauce.

DESSERT
Apple crumble

TO DRINK
Mu or Twig or Green tea.

Recipes

MUESLI BASE
Can be bought as a ready-mixed preparation of about five stone-ground whole cereals.

BROWN RICE
Should be cooked with care. May be short or long grain. Wash, boil and simmer in an enamel pot for about 45 minutes, until the ends of the grains pop, using 2 to 1 water to rice, and sea-salt to flavour.

RICE BALLS
Using a core of cooked seaweed or an umeboshi plum (from grain shops, Japanese shops, macrobiotic suppliers) wrap well-cooked cold brown rice around it to form a ball about the size of a golf ball. Deep-fry in sunflower oil or safflower oil until golden brown and crisp on the outside. May be eaten cold instead of sandwiches.

TEMPURA

Basically, any seasonal green or root vegetable dipped in buckwheat flour batter (made with water, not milk) and deep fried in sunflower or safflower oil.

Fish may also be prepared in this way, in smallish portions. Watercress sounds unlikely, but is delicious.

MISO STEW

Miso is a preparation of fermented soya beans, quite strong in flavour, so use with care. Add about a dessertspoonful of miso (a rich source of protein and vitamin B) to a mixed winter vegetable stew containing rice or lentils but no potatoes, tomatoes or aubergines.

UNLEAVENED BREAD

May be taken with all meals, using polyunsaturated margarine (no jams!).

Freshly ground wholewheat may be used, and the bread mix will prove naturally. Can be obtained ready-made from good delicatessens and grocery chain stores.

APPLE CRUMBLE

Cut the apples, add currants or raisins to sweeten, lightly stew, place in a casserole dish and top with flaked oatmeal or muesli bound with sunflower oil. Cook in a medium oven, 180°C/350°F (Gas Mark 4) until crisp on top.

Do not use tomatoes, potatoes, aubergines, citrus fruits or fruit juices, milk, meat or fowl, sugar, honey, coffee, alcohol, refined cereals. Various other recipes can be found in macrobiotic cookery books.

HYPO-ALLERGENIC DIET

If allergy is suspected as being the cause of cystitis, a very simple, bland diet should be followed for six days, to allow the system to eliminate all traces of the allergen. Then gradually introduce the foods you are used to eating, checking the pulse rate before and after eating or drinking. If, say, a salad produced an elevated pulse and, quite possibly, a sudden onset of symptoms, you must then test each ingredient of the salad singly. The most likely culprit would be a dressing, then possibly tomatoes, radishes, carrots or beetroot.

Food allergies are most commonly related to

- meat
- seafood
- dairy products
- coffee
- alcohol
- gluten (in wheat products)
- refined sugar
- yeast

Therefore, in our 'hypo-allergenic' regime these must all be avoided. Doctors specializing in dietary allergy tend to use extreme diets for the six-day period, such as lamb and pears only. There is no real way round this problem of utter boredom with food for a week unless you treat your mono-diet as an exciting and challenging way of achieving a high level of health and well-being, in a dramatically short time. Even if you do not have an actual food allergy, the semi-fast or mono-diet allows the body to carry out a thorough spring-cleaning.

During the first few days you will probably feel absolutely awful, because the blood is suddenly laden with toxic products released from storage tissues, which have to be processed and excreted by the liver and kidneys. Typically, on the first and second days there will be a heavy, throbbing frontal headache, on the second or third day a bruised feeling around the kidney area of the back and very concentrated pungent urine. At this time the cystitis is likely to be severe for a few hours, but should clear up quickly and cleanly. By the third or fourth day you will feel physically a bit weak, but probably have a feeling of mental clarity and sensitivity which is quite amazing to anyone who has not fasted before.

Hunger now starts showing its head, but must be resisted. Obviously, no strenuous activity, mental or physical, should be undertaken, as there is insufficient energy to cope. Stick it out until the morning of the seventh day, when you expand your intake with the alkaline-producing diet shown below. Try to eat things separately or in small mixtures, to simplify any detective work needed with your pulse test, which you now start.

Should the alkaline foods all prove innocent, move on to your normal diet, when any remaining allergies will become apparent. The guilty foods will henceforth have to be avoided unless you have special treatment with homoeopathic preparations of the foods, which will desensitize you.

I have found that the majority of patients coming to me with allergy problems respond best to cranial osteopathy, complemented by spinal osteopathy. This reduces stresses in the central nervous system which often predispose to allergic reaction. A visit to a cranial osteopath, or an applied kinesiologist, is well worth while as once any disorders in this area are rectified the tendency to allergy often disappears.

The Basic Diet

IN SPRING OR SUMMER
Freshly made yogurt and lettuce. Half a cupful of yogurt (preferably goats' milk) with a few lettuce leaves at normal mealtimes. One pear daily. Bottled, pure mineral water.

IN AUTUMN OR WINTER
Boiled brown rice, flavoured with sea-salt only *or* grapes and pure grape juice with no addivities. Bottled pure mineral water.

ALKALINE-PRODUCING (YIN) DIET

In Oriental terms, this diet is the opposite of the previous Yang diet, and it is the more generally indicated one for cystitis sufferers, as amply explained in earlier chapters. Basically, there is a predominance of fruit and vegetable foods, a regime advocated by most naturopathic writers this century. There can be dangers in taking it to extremes, however. Some people, such as hypoglycaemia sufferers, cannot tolerate the shortage of first-class protein. So if you should feel weak or emotionally unstable after a couple of weeks of this diet, you should obtain professional advice about your own individual dietary needs.

Within the confines of the foods listed, many varied and appetizing meals can be created, and you need not get bored. This diet should be followed until you are satisfied that all the symptoms have completely gone – so it may be a long-term thing. Try not to think of it as a diet, but rather as a healthy, normal way of eating.

Cabbage	Brazil nuts	Apples
Kale	Almonds	Pears
Lettuce	Swedes	Peaches
Cress	Turnips	Cherries
Watercress	Tomatoes	Pineapple
Celery	Beans	Grapefruit
Radishes	(fresh and dried)	Bananas
Courgettes	Carrots	
Cucumbers	Olives	
	Potatoes	
	Aubergines	

These foods should be balanced with a few acid-reaction foods. For instance:
Wholewheat bread or Pumpernickel (2 slices per day)
Cheese (average 2 oz/50g per day)
Eggs (average 3 per week)

Brown rice (in small quantities)
Muesli base (2 dessertspoonsful per day)

Suggested Menu

BREAKFAST
Soak 2 dessertspoonsful of muesli base in the same
  quantity of water overnight. Add freshly chopped or
  grated mixed fruits and nuts in the morning, squeeze
  the juice from a slice of lemon over it and add a little
  milk or yogurt.
A glass of weak lemon tea or a tisane.

MID-MORNING
Lemon tea or tisane.

LUNCH
A fresh mixed salad, with bread and honey if desired.

MID-AFTERNOON
Lemon tea or tisane.

EVENING MEAL
Cooked seasonal vegetables, preferably lightly steamed.
A potato in its jacket or brown rice.
A little cheese or egg – perhaps in a vegetable casserole.
Or a small helping of nut roast.
Fresh fruit salad.

ON RETIRING
Peppermint or elderflower and peppermint tea.

CHAPTER FIVE

A Balanced Way of Eating

When all your symptoms have cleared to your satisfaction, there is absolutely no point in going back to your old living habits, because those are what created the situation in the first place. We all have our own individual needs and preferences, and therefore the suggestions given here are in fairly general terms.

You will find that some of the more popular foods have been specifically omitted. However, if your favourites are missing, you will probably find that if you have already followed one of the previous remedial diets, your body will rebel should you try them.

There are good reasons for this – for instance, a bacon rasher will lie in the stomach for up to eleven hours after being eaten, causing excessive activity of the gastric juices; coffee constricts the blood vessels at the same time as it irritates the heart and nervous system. Now that your body has become cleaner and more balanced, it reacts violently to such substances.

Listen to what your body tells you. If you feel stodgy, breathless or nervy after a meal, think about what you had. Say you have eaten in a restaurant and had an omelette with vegetables and chips, fruit salad and coffee, and you feel peculiar. The first indiscretion has been the chips – lifeless starch and water resurrected from the deep freeze in heavily processed oil.

These will throw the stomach into overdrive, and the caffeine in the coffee will starve it of the blood it needs to cope with the situation. An after-dinner cigarette would make the problem even worse, as it would further constrict the blood vessels. The fruit would lie on top of the slowly digesting fried food, start to ferment and cause wind.

So let us try again. This time we have a fruit *hors d'oeuvre* – a melon for instance – the omelette with a boiled or baked potato and vegetable, a little cheese to follow, and a leisurely cup of tea at least ten minutes after finishing your food – after all, you do not want to dilute your digestive juices just as they are at the peak of their activity.

If you eat correctly 90 per cent of the time, your body will cope with a 10 per cent bending of the rules. It will probably let you know that it is a bit unhappy after an excessive meal, but that is a healthy sign, and means that your senses have not been blunted. You do not have to appear to be a total crank to stay healthy!

FOOD REFORM DIET

Approximately 50 per cent of your food intake should come from each column.

Lettuce
Carrots
Turnips
Beetroot
Swedes
Celery
Watercress
Radishes
Beans
Peas
Almonds
Brazils
All fresh fruits
All dried fruits
Potatoes
  (baked in jackets)

Beef
Lamb
Fish
Fowl
Unpolished (brown) rice
Wholemeal bread and
  other products
Cheese
Eggs
Buckwheat
Millet
Oatmeal
Butter
Margarine

Restricted Foods

TOMATOES, POTATOES, AUBERGINES
Very Yin, have them seldom, especially in winter.

REFINED FLOUR AND SUGAR
Special occasions only.

ALCOHOL
A little dry white wine can usually be tolerated.

COFFEE
Decaffeinated only. Do not drink too much as the chemicals used in the decaffeination process can be harmful.

RED MEAT
Lean, not more than two or three times a week. If you feel happy without it leave it out completely.

MILK
Many people are allergic to cow's milk. It is highly mucus-forming, and excessively Yin. Use only on muesli or in tea.

CONDIMENTS
Use sparingly. Avoid very rich dressings.

Forbidden Foods

BACON, PORK AND PORK PRODUCTS
Very difficult to digest and usually chemically adulterated.

CONVENIENCE FOODS IN GENERAL
Lack vitality, have many unhealthy additives and are generally denatured.

ICE-CREAM
Too cold for people with kidney/bladder difficulties and usually junk anyway.

CHAPTER SIX

Other Ways to Help Yourself

EXERCISES

To Correct Uterine Displacement

This exercise, performed regularly, will help to tip the uterus back and up, off the bladder.

Lie on your back on the floor, knees bent. Practice breathing with the diaphragm, one hand on your stomach, the other on your chest. Breathe down into your abdomen so that your lower hand rises on the inward breath. Let it release and try again until you are able to control the diaphragm well enough to breathe confidently in this way without hesitation. The ribs should be relatively immobile.

Now take a deep 'tummy' breath and, as you release it, straighten the hips so that the back rises off the floor and your body forms a straight line from shoulders to knees. As you take your next breath, allow the body to gently return to the floor, and repeat this twenty times morning and evening.

It is important that the breathing is done as described because the diaphragm, which is often virtually unused in women, is a pump which creates negative pressure in the abdomen as it lifts, therefore lifting the contents as well as pumping blood back from the legs and pelvis to the heart. Do not confine your diaphragm breathing to the exercises, everyone should do it all the time.

To Strengthen Abdomen

Lie on the floor on your back, take a deep breath and let it out slowly as you raise one leg to 45°. Count to three, then breathe in again as you slowly lower it. Repeat this five times with each leg alternately, and gradually increase the number of lifts as your muscles strengthen.

Now stretch your arms forwards towards your feet, raise the head to look forwards and roll the body up to a sitting position, as if to touch your toes. Stretch the arms forwards towards the toes, looking straight ahead, not bowing the head. Slowly unwind again on the floor, as if you were a carpet being rolled out, keeping the arms stretched toward the feet.

Repeat for as many times as you feel comfortable.

HYGIENE

This section will be considered rather obvious by most, but its importance is critical and the recommendations should be carefully followed.

The Importance of Air . . .

The infective organisms which normally cause cystitis are 'anaerobic', that is, they are killed by fresh air. They thrive in moist, warm, airless environments, the anal and vaginal areas being ideal for this. There is a perfectly normal colony of E Coli bacteria in the bowel which is essential to health, but it becomes a menace when it gets out! It only has a small bridge to cross should it find itself exposed, however, and it will migrate across the inch or so of moist, warm perineum to the vagina and a warm refuge as quickly as possible.

This bridge can be defended in a number of ways. The most obvious is air. Thus one should wear loose-fitting natural fibre clothing which will waft air through the area continuously. Tights, nylon briefs and 'all-in-ones' must be avoided at all times by the susceptible person. Then we can make the surface of the bridge most unsafe, by creating an alkaline environment. The E Coli needs an acid medium to survive, so alkaline-producing foods are the key to your 'internal' hygiene.

. . . and Water

Hosing down, especially with cold water, will of course tend to wash away the unwelcome guests, but all washing should be done with care because the skin in this area is quite delicate and easily irritated. Should the pores become damaged the bacteria will have lots of lovely footholds for their journey. Particularly, antiseptics, deodorants, talcs and perfumed soaps should be avoided. Many supposedly soothing and antiseptic preparations include the chemical hexachlorophene which is especially damaging. It can be found in shampoos and other toiletries, so do not wash your hair in the bath unless you are sure what you are using is innocent.

On finishing a bath, which should not be too hot, always splash or shower some cold fresh water around the genital area. It will stimulate local blood flow and drainage as well as washing away soap deposits from the pores. If you suffer from a chronic cystitis, it may well be worth having a bidet installed, which will play a fountain of clean water over the perineal area after every evacuation.

While all clothing must obviously be kept scrupulously clean, it is better to avoid detergent washing powders. Make sure, though, that every last bit of soap is thoroughly rinsed out of the material before drying.

Internal tampons are not usually a good idea for cystitis sufferers, as they tend to dry up the vaginal membranes and can cause irritation.

Douching, very popular in Europe, has never been widely used in Britain, but is a most effective way of cleansing the vaginal area and stimulating blood flow and drainage. It can be done with a bidet, or with a simple kit available from chemists. About once a week is enough, the area should not be scoured of its natural secretions too frequently.

DEALING WITH AN ACUTE ATTACK

1 Above all do not panic! Managed as described, the attack will be under control in the least possible time. 'Where the mind goes the body follows' – so think positively.

2 Drink a pint (575ml) of water.

3 Have a teaspoonful of bicarbonate of soda washed down with water or cordial. Repeat in a couple of hours.

4 Sip unchilled water frequently; have some parsley tea hourly.

5 Curl up with a hot water bottle on the tummy for five minutes or so, then alternate with cold wet towel.

6 Do not eat at all while the attack is acute.

7 If the body temperature rises above 100°F (37.8°C), apply a cold waist compress, as described below. If the temperature reaches 103°F (39.4°C), use a large compress from armpit to groin.

8 Gently rinse and dab dry the external genital area every time you have passed water. Apply a little vitamin E and calendula cream to the skin in the area to soothe it and discourage infection.

9 As the discomfort eases, cut down on liquid intake. Continued heavy drinking may upset the electrolyte balance.

COMPRESSES

Perhaps the most valuable naturopathic procedure next to diet control, compresses (or 'packs' as they are often known) are of tremendous help to the cystitis sufferer. They work by encouraging blood to race through the abdomen, and its internal organs, in order to carry away the excess heat or cold applied, and thus raise the level of cell nourishment and drainage, and assist the body's phagocytic (infection-fighting) activity.

They are so simple that many people just do not take them seriously; but the fact is that they will control almost any high temperature while assisting, not hindering, the body's recovery. Do not reach for the aspirin bottle, compresses will do a much better job in almost every case where such a thing might be considered.

Hot Packs

These are used to warm the body when it has become cold and devitalized, as might happen in chronic illness or old age. They are also useful as a preliminary to cold compresses where there is acute pain or spasm.

The easiest way to make one is to rinse a thick towel in very hot water, wring it firmly, and wrap it tightly around the waist and groin covering with a blanket or another dry towel, then retire to bed. If necessary, hot water bottles can be used in addition. The compress should normally stay warm and so gradually dries out. Replace it if it becomes cold.

Cold Packs

Suitable for most reasonably active people, these cause an intense rush of blood to the area of application, which absorbs the cold and causes the compress to become hot. It therefore starts to steam and dries out within a few hours, acting as a poultice on the skin while doing so. This helps to clean the blood and tissues. (In the highly toxic body they can become noticeably stained from one application!)

Prepare a piece of cotton or linen cloth, such as from an old sheet, shirt etc., long enough to go once round your waist and about eight inches (20cm) deep (unless you are using a half body pack – then the depth of your trunk). Rinse it out in cold water, wring it firmly, shake it out and lay it on a warm woolly muffler, shawl or blanket. Have a couple of large safety pins ready to hold it in position. Get really warm – either with a hot bath or lots of bedclothes – quickly uncover yourself, wrap the compress round the middle, fasten it and dive under the bedclothes. The compress should become hot in about five to ten minutes – if it cools take it off, it must be too wet or you are too cold. With any luck it will send you off into a sound sleep within minutes, and when you wake it will be dry and can be removed or replaced.

It is obviously preferable to have someone else to do the preparation of these packs, to allow you to keep as calm and warm as possible. Do not use any analgesics while using cold packs – they are not only unnecessary, they may interfere with the body's response to the stimulus of the cold water.

Diagnostic Chart

Pain	Possible Cause
before period with intercourse	anteverted or prolapsed uterus or post-operative adhesions
after intercourse with bearing down feeling	prolapsed bladder
with walking with sitting	anteverted or prolapsed uterus or prolapsed bladder
when worried or excited away from home	emotional
after drinking alcohol with skin or other chronic symptoms	allergy
with fever back pain leg pain	ureter or kidney infection
after eating	constipation or post-operative adhesions or allergy
itching	pruritis (stress)
itching with discharge	thrush (antibiotics)
burning	local infection

Suitable Alternative Treatment	Diet
Exercise (see page 43) osteopathy, acupuncture	cleansing diet, then Yang, then food reform
osteopathy, acupuncture	Yang diet, then food reform
osteopathy, acupuncture	Yang diet, then food reform
counselling/psychotherapy acupuncture, homoeopathy	Yang diet, then food reform
homoeopathy	hypo-allergenic diet, then food reform
naturopathy, herbalism	fasting, then cleansing diet, then alkaline diet, then food reform
kinesiology, naturopathy, acupuncture, cranial osteopathy	cleansing or hypo-allergenic diets, food reform
counselling/psychotherapy	food reform
stop antibiotics	vitamins A and E, food reform, acidophillus tablets
naturopathy, acupuncture, herbalism	cleansing diet, alkaline diet, food reform

Index

Also available:

Diets to help
ASTHMA AND HAY FEVER
Suitable for all catarrhal conditions

Roger Newman Turner

Asthma and hay fever can be made worse by eating certain foods, but there are also nutritional guidelines that you can follow to help *manage* the condition. This book explains:

- why some people are prone to asthma or hay fever
- how to cut down on mucus-forming foods
- how to increase your intake of protective vitamins and minerals

It includes basic diets to help control the condition and specific diets for more acute symptoms.

ROGER NEWMAN TURNER is a leading naturopath, osteopath and acupuncturist. He has many years' experience treating a wide range of conditions and runs practices in Harley Street, London and Letchworth, Hertfordshire.

Diets to help
GLUTEN AND WHEAT ALLERGY

Suitable for those with coeliac disease

Rita Greer

Here is sound practical advice on gluten allergy, wheat sensitivity and coeliac disease. It explains:

- what gluten is
- the symptoms of allergy
- a list of 'safe' foods and those to avoid
- useful alternatives to wheat, rye, barley and oats

Also included are basic recipes, emergency menus and facts about coeliac disease.

RITA GREER is an experienced diet therapist and cookery writer. She has many years' experience of coping with a gluten-free diet.

DIETS TO HELP ARTHRITIS	0 7225 1730 0	£2.99	☐
DIETS TO HELP ASTHMA AND HAY FEVER	0 7225 2911 2	£2.99	☐
DIETS TO HELP COLITIS	0 7225 1704 1	£2.99	☐
DIETS TO HELP CONTROL CHOLESTEROL	0 7225 1757 2	£2.99	☐
DIETS TO HELP DIABETES	0 7225 1731 9	£2.99	☐
DIETS TO HELP MULTIPLE SCLEROSIS	0 7225 2389 0	£2.99	☐
DIETS TO HELP GLUTEN AND WHEAT ALLERGY	0 7225 2910 4	£2.99	☐
DIETS TO HELP PSORIASIS	0 7225 2929 5	£2.99	☐

All these books are available from your local bookseller or can be ordered direct from the publishers.

To order direct just tick the titles you want and fill in the form below:

Name: _____

Address: _____

_____

_____ Postcode: _____

Send to: Thorsons Mail Order, Dept 3, HarperCollins*Publishers*, Westerhill Road, Bishopbriggs, Glasgow G64 2QT.
Please enclose a cheque or postal order or your authority to debit your Visa/Access account —

Credit card no: _____

Expiry date: _____

Signature: _____

— up to the value of the cover price plus:
UK & BFPO: Add £1.00 for the first book and 25p for each additional book ordered.
Overseas orders including Eire: Please add £2.95 service charge. Books will be sent by surface mail but quotes for airmail despatches will be given on request.

24 HOUR TELEPHONE ORDERING SERVICE FOR ACCESS/VISA CARDHOLDERS — TEL: **041 772 2281.**